END BEDWETTING NOW

**NO PILLS! NO EQUIPMENT! NO COST!
A SCIENCE-BASED, MEDICALLY
PROVEN WAY TO STOP UNWANTED
PEEING AND POOPING**

**PROFESSOR ANGEL GARCIA-FERNANDEZ
PROFESSOR PETER PETROS
WITH ALAN GOLD**

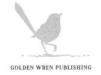

GOLDEN WREN PUBLISHING

First published in 2019 by Golden Wren Publishing Ltd. Sydney, Australia.

© Golden Wren Publishing Ltd.

The moral rights of the author have been asserted.

Title: End Bedwetting Now; A truly simple and effective way to stop children wetting their beds.

Paperback ISBN: 978-0-6487102-2-6
EBook ISBN: 978-0-6487102-7-1

Subject: Self-Help

All enquiries should be made to the publisher at:
rebecca@goldenwrenpublishing.com

This book is of a general nature, and no information is intended to be construed as professional medical advice. It does not take into account your individual health, medical, physical or emotional situation or needs. It deals solely with the issue of certain pelvic floor muscles, and is NOT a substitute for proper medical attention, treatment, examination, advice, treatment of existing conditions or diagnosis and is not intended to provide a clinical diagnosis nor take the place of proper medical advice from a fully qualified medical practitioner.

www.goldenwrenpublishing.com

AN ENCOURAGING INTRODUCTION TO A DIFFICULT TOPIC

Bedwetting in youngsters, as well as incontinence in grown-ups, is an enormous global health problem, affecting hundreds of millions of people.

It causes shame and social isolation, profound embarrassment and feelings of disgrace and inferiority in sufferers. Yet despite the havoc which serious bedwetting and incontinence can cause in its victims, it's one which men, women and children are often forced to suffer with in silence.

The effects of occasional, or frequent, bedwetting or incontinence on people often changes their lifestyles, and, unlike other ailments, is invariably born alone, in segregation, it's victims largely hidden from society because of the humiliation and awkwardness it causes sufferers. In the case of children, bed wetting long after they should have stopped wearing nappies, even into their teens, can cause serious psychological and personality problems which may last long into adulthood.

Yet instead of this being a publicly discussed social issue, incontinence is a hushed-up global pandemic which causes enormous personal distress, solitude and emotional damage, to say nothing of the financial cost, time wasted undergoing useless tests, and expensive visits to doctors. Virtually every doctor on earth will tell sufferers that there's little which can be done to cure incontinence in adults other than to wear pads; that bed wetting in children is usually a 'phase' they'll grow out of; and only changes in a child's lifestyle can reduce his or her bedwetting. And all of these pearls of wisdom and other old wives tales, are wrong! Totally wrong!

And the harm which is done by these antiquated and incorrect assumptions and obsolete medical conventions, is incalculable. Millions upon millions of kids growing up, and nearly a billion – yes, a billion – women who agonize with incontinence, will continue to suffer while doctors remain unaware of, and untrained in, recent research into one of the most important yet least understood parts of the human body...the pelvic floor. It's true! Almost no doctors, trained by the very best university hospitals, are aware of recent ground-breaking medical research which has uncovered how a person's pelvic floor actually works! That's why we Professors of Medicine have written this book. We want to put this knowledge into the hands of mothers and fathers, men and women, so that if doctors can't help you cure your children of bed wetting, YOU will now be able to.

We have applied the same revolutionary methodology behind the 5,000,000 women successfully cured of one form of incontinence, urinary stress, designed to strengthen the collagen in the ligaments, without any surgery, only asking sufferers to regularly do easy-to-perform exercises of key pelvic floor muscles.

This book puts into the hands of parents, grandparents and carers, a simple, elegant method which, for the first time in history, will enable them to understand, and help to cure their child's bedwetting.

The academic paper on which this book is based and which was published by a leading medical journal, can be found at the back of this book. Your doctor might be interested in reading it.

MEET THE AUTHORS

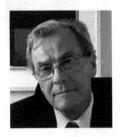

PROFESSOR ANGEL GARCIA FERNANDEZ

Professor Angel Garcia Fernandez MD PhD has been the Chief Professor of Medicine and Surgery, specializing in Child Urology at the National University of Cordoba and the Chef de Clinic of the Necker-Enfants Malades Hospital of the University of René Descartes, University of Paris, France. He has been the Specialist Pediatric Surgeon of the Argentine Society of Childhood Surgery since December, 1980.

Professor Garcia Fernandez has written numerous peer-reviewed periodicals and is a founding member of publications for national and international academic and professional books at Sociedad IberoAmerican de Urologia Infantil, and founding member of the Latin American Pelvic Floor Association, a Member of the French Association of Urologia and a Member of the International Children's Continence Society.

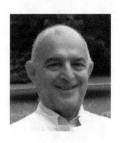

PROFESSOR PETER PETROS

Professor Peter Petros, DSc DS (UWA) PhD (Uppsala) MB BS MD (Syd) FRCOG (Lond) is a highly experienced pelvic floor reconstructive surgeon. He is internationally recognized as a leader in the field of incontinence and prolapse both in basic science and surgery. In the early 1990s, he and the late Professor Ulf Ulmsten from the University of Uppsala, Sweden, wrote a 79 page description of the Integral Theory of Female Urinary Incontinence which stated that stress urinary incontinence and what is now known as 'overactive bladder' did not originate from the bladder itself, but from looseness in the supporting ligaments of the urethra and vagina.

The reason for the looseness was deficient collagen in the ligaments. Two years prior to this publication, Petros and John Papadimitriou, both from the Royal Perth Hospital invented a new surgical method, how to create a new collagenous ligament using a tape implanted in the exact position of the damaged ligament. This was the basis for the midurethral sling operation for cure of urinary stress incontinence.

More than 5,000,000 such operations have been performed between 1996 and 2018. Since 1993, the Theory has evolved into a complete system of management as the Integral Theory System (ITS), which is not only a method of surgery, but also special non-surgical methods which can strengthen the automatic muscles and ligaments of the female pelvis. It is this part of the ITS which has been applied to cure children with bedwetting.

Professor Petros has authored more than 250 original scientific articles on incontinence and prolapse, has been awarded 4 doctorates and has written a major medical textbook on 'The Female Pelvic Floor' now in its 3rd edition, which has been printed in 10 languages.

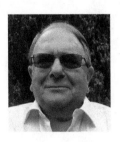

ALAN GOLD

Alan Gold has written over 30 books, both fiction and non-fiction. He became interested in medical scandals concerning incontinence and chronic pelvic pain in 2014. Alan has spent the past 5 years intensively investigating every aspect of the incontinence story, the mesh controversies, why the most recent discoveries in the understanding of the pelvic floor aren't taught in medical schools, as well as the pervasive influence of the $35 billion p.a. drug industry.

He uncovered disturbing evidence that women are being told by existing experts in the field that cures for bladder, bowel and chronic pain problems is not available. They ARE! As are cures for bed wetting. When Alan heard of the early results from the bed wetting studies, he, like the two Professors of Medicine who have authored this book, had some difficulty in understanding how such a simple method as exercises could possibly have so profound an effect.

As it happened, one of his colleagues had a 10-year old son with a severe bed wetting problem. After discussions with Professor Petros, Alan suggested the child do the required exercises every morning and every night. It was, after all, minimally invasive and the child's mother had nothing to lose.

Remarkably, the child became dry within one week and with regular exercises, has stayed dry since. This gave Alan a strong incentive to persuade the authors that they should make their discoveries known to the world at large. As an internationally published and translated novelist and opinion columnist, Alan has assisted Professors Petros and Garcia Fernandez with the book's structure, planning and content.

CONTENTS

BEDWETTING –
JUST DON'T BLAME THE KIDS

It's a pain for their parents but a nightmare for their children.

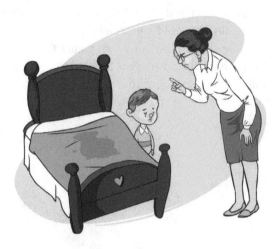

Childhood should be...but for around 15% of our kids, tragically isn't...a time of joy and pleasure. As kids' brains develop, once they're walking and talking, it's a time of learning, to socialize with other children, to play, to discover new things, and to be an important part of the family and especially their immediate play group.

Pre-school, Kindergarten, Elementary are usually the start of our children's process of proper socializing, where they befriend others, form little cliques and understand the rules and regulations of obeying the instructions of their teachers.

The majority of children are able to transition from the security and intimacy of a one-on-one relationship with their parents and siblings, to the group dynamics of pre-school, kindergarten and then their first experience of formal school education.

But there's a significant number of kids who don't fit into this pattern, and who either exclude themselves from the group, or are excluded from the group for no fault of theirs. These are the bed wetters, boys and girls no longer in nappies, but who can't seem to control their bladders or bowels, and the results are wet and smelly clothes, tears of embarrassment, and cries for help. And the end result is often social exclusion, ridicule, and isolation. No sleepovers, no going to grandparent's homes or friends' houses, and in severe cases, no going to movies or parties or concerts. This is especially embarrassing when children grow older and should be increasingly independent of the home, yet still can't control their problem.

And what kid aged five or six or seven wants to stay at a friend's house when he or she is forced to wear a protective pad at night time or suffer the humiliation of waking up in the morning and having to tell the friend's parents that he or she has wet the bed?

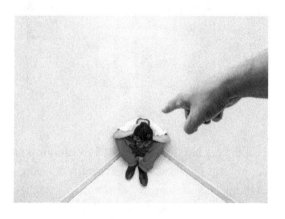

It even affects sport. If youngsters aged from five upwards are still wearing anti-soiling protection, a bit like nappies, then they're severely embarrassed when changing for sport at school or on weekends.

These bed wetting children can be aged from just three years of age, up to their late teens. And in some severe cases, involuntary bedwetting can persist even when a person is in his or her 20's, 30's and even 40's.

For hundreds of years, bed wetters have been blamed as the cause of their own problems. They're told – by parents or teachers or friends – that they're soiling their clothes or bed sheets because they're careless, or they've drunk too much at night, or they're forgetful, or they just don't care, or that they're a nuisance and should grow up…and worst of all, they're punished, exiled from friends and family and classmates, and told to learn how to hold on.

All that this condemnation does is compound the misery these poor kids are already suffering. By sheeting the blame back to the sufferer, the guilt feelings can become deeply rooted in the child's psyche and can cause long-term adverse effects when the kids grow up.

And it's ALL SO UNNECESSARY. IT ISN'T THEIR FAULT!

Why? Because there is a cure for bed wetting.

Yes...a cure!

Treatments in the past have involved drinking less liquid at night so as not to fill the bladder; or alarms attached to the sheet which ring and wake the poor kid up the moment he or she begins to pee, or worst of all, pills which act on the child's pituitary gland in the brain, with potentially harmful consequences. Then there are expensive and useless sessions with a psychiatrist or psychologist so that the kid will 'learn' not to pee at night, or how to 'hold on' until he or she reaches the toilet.

The results of all of this mumbo-jumbo medical nonsense is so marginal, so negligible and so damaging to the child's self-confidence, that the expense on the parents and the psychological pressure on the child, are just not worth it.

Without doctors, pills, surgery
and at no cost whatsoever

It's not often in medicine that a genuine, life-changing breakthrough occurs, but one has recently happened in the field of adult incontinence, and now this amazing breakthrough has been extended to cure bed wetting in children.

This breakthrough in understanding the cause of bed wetting, and its cure, is so incredible, so life-affirming, that tens of millions of children (and many adults) around the world will be able to cure themselves of involuntary bowel or bladder leakages.

The most recent studies of bed wetting has found conclusively that the problem has NOTHING to do with the bladder or the children's brains, or their laziness or unwillingness to learn.

It's due to a simple MECHANICAL cause within the body. And the cure is perhaps the simplest cure imaginable. The treatment, which our own university studies have shown is totally effective in up to 80% of cases, is:

- Not surgical, or requiring pills or potions
- Not reducing liquid at night; it has NOTHING to do with the bladder
- Not requiring electronic monitoring or other bells or whistles
- Not psychiatry or psychotherapy
...and certainly NOT punishment

THE CURE IS EXERCISE

Yes, you read that correctly. If a child does the right exercises to strengthen some of the muscles in his or her pelvic floor, then bedwetting and accidental wetting during the day, or whilst playing sport, will almost certainly disappear.

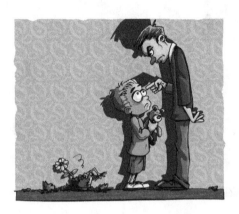

It was proven by Professor Angel Garcia Fernandez with 80% success in one of the hospital and university clinics where he currently works. Professor Garcia Fernandez was working in collaboration with Professor Peter Petros, whose revolutionary investigations into the working of the female pelvic floor, led him to believe that it was either poor ligament, or poor muscle development, which were the cause of children wetting their beds. And that the muscles can be strengthened by exercise.

Although all children's activities and natural play are excellent, certain key muscles of the pelvic floor may be under-exercised and need strengthening.

STOP PRESS

We even have experience of a 17-year-old boy who wet his bed, and through exercises, has now stopped. Why is he special? Because this lad was a top class rugby football player. His body was a machine. Strong, good looking and incredibly healthy. His muscles were at peak condition. Yet no exercises he did for his sport conditioned his pelvic floor muscles. But when he did OUR exercises, he stopped bedwetting in a week AND HAS REMAINED DRY EVER SINCE.

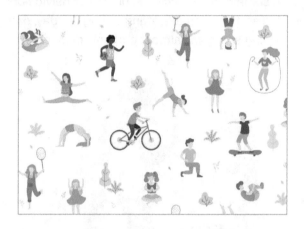

It was an AMAZING cure. And proof that what we're doing is effective.

Based on Professor Petros' research into adult incontinence, Professor Garcia Fernandez instituted a research study in his University Hospital in Argentina.

Children who wet their beds at night were brought to him and he conducted a scientific study. First, he divided the children into two groups.

The first group he told the mothers and fathers to encourage and monitor their children to do a simple exercise every morning and every night for a month in order to strengthen specific muscles in the child's pelvic floor, muscles which the body uses to open and close the waste tubes of the bladder and bowel.

In the second group the children were given a harmless placebo pill to take and were told that this could help them but were NOT told to do the exercises.

After a matter of weeks, the placebo pill regimen was stopped for ethical reasons...because the kids taking the pills showed no improvement, but the kids performing the morning and night exercise showed dramatic improvements. So, the group who were taking the placebo were then instructed to undertake the simple exercises for two minutes, morning and night as the other children were.

CORE ELEMENTS OF TREATMENT FOR BEDWETTING

It is important to realise that this cure depends on exercising muscles in a person's pelvic area. Muscles must be exercised to gain their maximum effectiveness. Please understand, these diagrams represent a strictly summarised core of the program, and to achieve the best results psychologically and physically for your children, you will need to read the rest of this book.

1. Squatting 10-15 times morning and evening without fail for 4 months and continue afterwards.
2. The child must be supervised by a parent who keeps a diary.
3. Encourage the child to do all his/her activities by squatting on the floor.

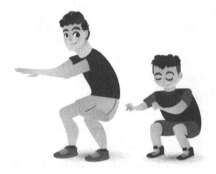

Squatting exercise. Begin standing and descend to this position.

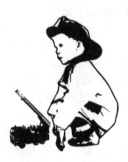

Encourage the child to do all activitie squatting on the floor

AND THE RESULTS?
AMAZING...READ ON...

Another month later, the parents and kids returned with huge smiles on their faces. In the vast majority of the children, they were sleeping dry through the night.

No wet PJs, no wet bed sheets, no sodden blankets, and no tears. And during the day, the children reported no accidents, no embarrassment and a normal day at school, trauma and humiliation free.

Yes! All it took was squatting exercises. It was that simple.

Specific exercises of particular muscles in the pelvic floor of children will cure bed wetting. These are exercises which kids can carry out at home, exercises which can be turned into games that they'll enjoy, exercises which are so simple, they require NO equipment, can be done in front of the television before and after school and which will stop bed wetting in around a couple of months.

But how can exercises for incontinence work for children when it is well known that they don't work so well in older adults, especially women who are post-menopausal?

There are two answers to this question. The first answer takes us back to 1990, when a major discovery was made by Professor Petros on how the bladder works which was published for the first time. The simple answer is that existing exercises, usually taught to mothers who had just given birth, unfortunately train the wrong muscle, a muscle called the 'Kegel muscle'. However, realizing that Kegel exercises had virtually no influence on incontinence, different pelvic muscle exercises were developed by a colleague of Professor Petros, Dr. Patricia Skilling, and were designed to train the three key muscles which open and close the waste tubes. This mechanism was discovered by Professor Petros and the late Professor Ulf Ulmsten of Uppsala University and gynecologist to the Swedish Royal Family.

These 3 muscles automatically contract against the pelvic ligaments to keep the urethral tube closed to stop the flow, or open to urinate. Exactly the same muscles that control the bowel. If the ligaments are loose, the bladder and bowel tubes can't be closed, so urine and feces can leak out. Also, depending on which ligaments are loose, the tubes can't be opened, so children have bladder emptying problems or are constipated.

The second answer is to do with age and collagen – more about collagen later in this book. Exercises hardly work in older, post-menopausal women as they are in a collagen-loss mode. Young children are in full-steam ahead collagen formation mode to strengthen and reinforce tissues, ligaments and bones. When the 3 muscles pull against the ligaments, they strengthen them, much as an athlete strengthens the sinews of their muscles when they train.

As stated above, the cause of bed wetting in children and adults is because key muscles and ligaments of a person's pelvis are under-developed, and simple 2-minute exercises, performed every morning and every night, has been shown to completely cure bed wetting in as quickly as a month or two. Of course, the exercises have to be maintained, and the child needs to become more physically active in order to keep these ligaments strong and prevent the issue reoccurring again.

And that's what this book is all about. Showing you a simple, at-home, non-medical, non-surgical cure for bed wetting in children, teens, and adults. Yes! Adults, because exercising the pelvic floor is as important in preventing current, or future incontinence, as is exercising other muscles of the body. And it's especially important for all adult women to squat to pick up things from the ground, rather than bending over. Every time a woman squats, she exercises key muscles in her pelvis which will be important in future years to help prevent incontinence. So to ALL mums and dads...don't bend to pick up things from the floor...squat!

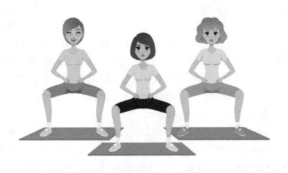

This cost-free exercise and medical 'treatment' – YES, YOU READ THAT CORRECTLY…COST-FREE TREATMENT – which can be done by any child or adult has been shown to be completely effective in up to 80% of the kids who were part of the study group conducted by Professor Garcia Fernandez at his major university hospital. The kids began the study still wetting their clothes, bed sheets and blankets, and after spending a couple of months doing the simple exercises, almost all of them had completely stopped. They were dry at night, in the morning, at school, at play and while watching television in the comfort of their homes.

The Cost to their parents? NIL
The Value to the Child? Incalculable

As you read on, you will learn how this book will vastly improve the lives and well-being of kids who can't control their bladders or bowels, we'll tell you why some youngsters and adults remain bed wetters, and why these natural exercises to strengthen muscles in the pelvic floor, actually work.

We'll tell you what exercises your children…well, all children… should be doing and which every woman in the world should also be doing to prevent the onset of incontinence in later life. A problem that adults are uneducated about, especially mothers who have given natural births. A problem that happens to the elderly who have not had a physically active lifestyle. A problem that will escalate because of the technology changing society that keeps children in a sitting position and inactive.

But if there's one thing which we hope this little book will prove conclusively, it's that kids who wet their beds at night, or who don't make it to the toilet during the day and who soil their clothes, are blameless. It's NOT their fault! Their ligaments need strengthening, they have muscles which need exercising, and then, in the vast majority of the cases, the problem will disappear, and their lives to be normal kids in a normal society, can resume.

These boys and girls need your help, as loving parents and peers. They're desperate for their problem to be solved. And all it takes is for one to participate in a daily exercise regime morning and night.

They need help! And now, help is in the hands of every mom and dad.

SO WHAT ACTUALLY CAUSES BED WETTING AND DAYTIME INCONTINENCE?

Thirty years ago, two highly qualified medical specialists, Professor Ulf Umsten from Sweden and the co-author of this book, Professor Peter Petros from Australia, worked collaboratively at Uppsala, one of the world's most prestigious university hospitals, and were researching adult incontinence in women.

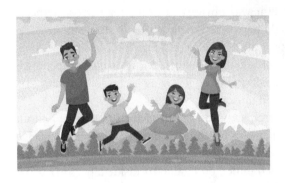

Professor Petros returned to his home country, where he later discovered the greatest breakthrough in women's health in 100 years. He found that it was the action of muscles acting on ligaments inside a woman's pelvis, which opened and closed the bladder and bowel waste tubes. His discovery flew in the face of two thousand years of the understanding of the human body, but when he applied his discovery to the treatment of a common condition of women – stress incontinence – which had until then been virtually incurable, his ideas of how the pelvic floor worked, were proven beyond doubt.

His operation has since been conducted with overwhelming success on five million women.

In conjunction with colleague, Dr. Patricia Skilling, a graduate from the University of St Andrews in Scotland, and Head of Pelvic Floor Rehabilitation in the Kvinno Centre Perth, Western Australia, they reasoned that if these same muscles in boys and girls could be strengthened, it would put an end to bed wetting and involuntary loss of urine and feces. His theories were tested by his Argentine collaborator, Professor Angel Garcia Fernandez, with prodigious success.

He simply noticed that one of his patients, a woman with constant urine leakage, stopped leaking when a particular ligament was supported with a finger placed immediately behind the pubic bone. Suddenly, her waste tube, her urethra, closed and the leakage stopped. When the tightening was released, the leakage continued. Again, he put pressure on the ligament to effectively shorten it, and the tube closed.

Suddenly it was obvious to Professor Petros...either the ligament which should have acted to close the urethra was stretched beyond its limits...like a piece of elastic which had been overextended...or the muscles which should have been acting on the ligament, were somehow too weak to act and close it. Or as he reasoned, both were connected and worked in unison.

His research showed that all of the knowledge and understanding of the human pelvis for the past hundreds of years, was INCORRECT!

So in reality, it was now proven beyond doubt that particular muscles **which pulled on ligaments** inside a person's pelvic floor, were responsible for opening and closing the bladder and the bowel.

This amazing discovery has been used in 5,000,000 successful operations which has cured women of stress incontinence, a particular type of leakage which often devastated the lifestyles of older people.

Professor Petros then determined that as the pelvic floor is fundamentally the same in adults and children, bed wetting and the inability to control the flow of urine and feces in children must be caused by under-developed ligaments which are not yet able to close the waste tubes. As will be seen later in the book, his views were influenced by many women in their early twenties who gave a history of having suffered bedwetting which did not clear up puberty and was only cured when the ligaments were surgically repaired using the tape method that was so successful for urinary stress incontinence.

And the Cure?

Exercise those particular muscles, and the problem will disappear. The now-famous publication by Professor Petros and his Swedish colleague Professor Ulmsten had uncovered the previously unknown ways in how the bladder stayed closed. Their discovery amazed the medical community, and also stirred up controversy among traditionalists who saw their life's work as being undermined.

But these discoveries couldn't be denied. Amazingly, incontinence in children and adults has NOTHING to do with the bladder. It only has to do with having strong ligaments against which the pelvic muscles could contract.

In older women, who couldn't control their bladder, the cure was to insert a tape to strengthen the ligament. This created new collagen which covered the tape, mimicking the way in which the body used to work.

And the same principle which has surgically cured 5,000,000 women of stress incontinence can NOW be applied in a **non-surgical** way to children who suffer from bedwetting, with scientifically reported cure rates of up to 80%.

In the early 2000's Professor Petros began working with Dr. Patricia Skilling, a St. Andrew's University educated physician. They reasoned that the same principle which surgically cured the women with stress incontinence, could be applied non-surgically in younger women.

Dr. Skilling devised a method of strengthening the natural pelvic floor closure muscles which work in an automatic way. The patient isn't even aware of the muscles contracting. Though few patients were 100% cured, Dr. Skilling achieved a remarkable success, from 50% to 90% improvement in some symptoms, for women with bladder, bowel and chronic pelvic pain problems, and chronic pelvic pain problems for which no cause could be found.

So why does what works in adults also cure bedwetting in children, a problem which is suffered by tens of millions of kids around the world, causing them profound embarrassment, and in severe cases, social isolation?

Go to any doctor about your child's bed wetting, and they'll tell you next-to-nothing about pelvic floor muscles. Instead, you'll be told that bed wetting is a problem of the bladder, and that your child has to drink less at night, or that your child sleeps 'too deeply' at night and loses 'control', or that an alarm is necessary to wake them the moment there's some moisture in the bed, or they'll have to take tablets which work on the pituitary gland (a potentially dangerous treatment in some cases)...or a myriad other old-wives tales. But none of these involve a cure; they're just inadequate and often incorrect treatments of the symptom. They don't do anything to treat the cause.

A SYMPTOM OF OUR CHILDREN'S MODERN LIFESTYLE?

Most children, of course, stop wetting their beds and their pajamas when they no longer need nappies, but still, about 15% of boys and girls aged five years and older continue to wet their beds.

The number decreases up to the age of 10, but even though the percentage is relatively small, the numbers of children who wet themselves at night, or during the day, is very significant...worldwide it numbers in the millions.

There really are no records in history to show whether bedwetting is a relatively recent phenomenon, or whether our ancestor's children suffered from the problem. We know anecdotally from our patients that many children with bedwetting problems had an adult near relative who suffered from the same problem. What we also know for certain is that bedwetting in youngsters and incontinence in grown-ups is an enormous global health problem, affecting hundreds of millions of people. As we've said, it causes social isolation, profound embarrassment and feelings of shame and inferiority in sufferers. Yet despite the havoc which serious bedwetting and incontinence can cause its victims, it's one which men, women and children suffer in silence.

The effects which occasional, or frequent, bedwetting or incontinence has on people often changes their lifestyles, and, unlike other ailments, is invariably borne alone, in segregation, it's victims largely hidden from society because of the shame and embarrassment it causes sufferers.

Yet instead of this being a publicly discussed social issue, incontinence is a pandemic which causes enormous personal distress, solitude and emotional damage, to say nothing of the financial cost, time wasted undergoing useless pathology tests such as urodynamics, and unnecessary visits to doctors. And anecdotally, bedwetting seems to be a growing phenomenon amongst children, certainly in the First World.

Perhaps...and this is ONLY speculation on our part...it's because today's kids aren't exercising as much as children in history. And if that's the case, and there's a growing body of evidence to show that it is, then we have to blame television, computers, smart phones, and other electronic devices.

Previous generations of children were always out and about, in the streets playing with their little friends, running and jumping and skipping and all the other games which kids play. They were riding their bikes to school and racing around the neighborhood. Suburban streets after school were full of the yells and laughter of local kids playing with each other in the road, marking hopscotch and cricket pitches on pavements, and quickly scurrying away at the sound of an oncoming car. The neighborhood parks were full of kids playing football, using bundles of clothes as goalposts. Walls of houses played the support for basketball hoops, driveways became run-ups for football nets and front yards were trampled underfoot as cricket pitches.

Oddly, these days, such frenetic after-school activities seem to be absent from most suburban streets. This most recent generation – our children and grandchildren – are much more sessile. In their early years, they ride little tricycles – presents from grandparents – around the house or up and down driveways – but when they're five or six, they're tending to park their bikes to gather dust in a garage, because instead of riding from place to place, mum and dad stick the kids in the back of the car, and drive them.

From an early age, when they come home from school, kids these days sit for hours watching television or on iPads, or with their mobile smart phones texting friends, or downloading all manner of stuff from their computers. Whereas in previous generations, suburban streets were full of groups and gangs and friends walking and running and playing it was hard to get the kids inside then, today residential streets are virtually empty after school. You just don't see kids playing games outdoors like they used to.

Again, we stress this is an observation, not based on any scientific research, but perhaps the lifestyle of kids...sitting instead of moving, being driven to places instead of walking...is causing the pelvic floor muscles to be under-developed, and not to function as Nature intended.

Perhaps...

THE WONDERFUL HIDDEN SECRET
IN ALL OF OUR BODIES

It's now time for us to introduce you to an amazing structure inside your body, and the body of every single human being, about which you probably know very little or can hardly remember from biology classes at school.

Say hello to...Collagen!

So, what's collagen? Well, think of a piece of steak cooking on the griddle. There's the muscle which is juicy and delicious; then there's the fat around the edge which should be eaten in moderation...and often there's a hard, white strip which is difficult to cut and almost impossible to chew known as sinew. That's a ligament, whose structure is composed of collagen.

This wonderful substance, collagen, is a natural part of the body's tissues. Collagen is the most abundant protein in the human body, and it's absolutely integral in building bones, muscles, skin and tendons. It holds the body together, a bit like the sub-structure inside a building to give strength and organization, and it's where the bricks, wood, and plaster are constructed.

In older men and women, collagen isn't produced nearly as much as it is in growing youngsters, which often accounts for the 'stoop' of old age and for diseases like osteoporosis. It leaches out of the body, and in women, this is especially a problem after menopause.

But in youngsters, collagen is there in abundance, and that's why their bodies are much more flexible than adults. Children and young adults are in collagen-production mode until the age of 20 or 21. As is well-known, when an athlete trains with weights, it strengthens the muscle, the ligament the muscles pull against, and even the bone itself.

Collagen 'coats' the ligament to strengthen it, and this is particularly important in the ligaments in the pelvis which control the opening and closing of the bladder and the bowel.

Which brings us back to the muscles. Imagine a tug-of-war. Two teams are lined up with a rope in between them; the intention is that when the rope is taut, one team will use its strength to pull the other team across the line, and win. The other team will resist and use its strength to pull the opposing team over to their side of the line.

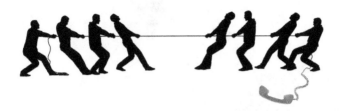

As you can see from this cartoon, two sets of muscles pull on a ligament, and the 'telephone' is the signaling mechanism of nerves which go to the brain and tell it to open and close the bladder or bowel when the need to pee or poo arises.

Think of it this way. Pulling on the taut rope (i.e. the ligament) from both sides keeps the bladder and bowel tightly shut.

When one team relaxes and stops pulling, the other team pulls them over the line, which is what happens to make the bladder or bowel open. But what happens if the ligament is loose? Then no matter how the muscles try to work, they won't be effective in opening and closing the waste tubes.

This isn't so much of a problem during the day, but the fact that a child is lying down in bed at night alters the geometry of the child's internal body organs, and it can become an issue.

During the day, the child is in the upright position. To illustrate the issue, we'll show you how it works in a girl in diagram 1.1.

The 3 muscles pull the vagina (blue) in opposite directions against the from ligaments (PUL) and the back ligaments (USL) to add tension to it.

This stretching supports the nerve endings 'N' which activate the emptying reflexes for the bladder and bowel (green arrow).

If the ligaments are weak, the muscles cannot stretch the bladder and bowel effectively. The nerve endings 'N' cannot be supported, so they send impulses (green arrows) to the brain cortex. If these impulses cannot be controlled by the brain cortex, the children cannot control the emptying and either wet or soil themselves.

DIAGRAM 1.1

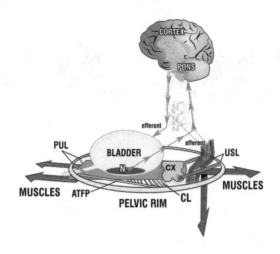

The cure for bedwetting in children had its beginnings in a casual conversation in March 2018, in a scientific meeting in Mexico City, in which South American pediatric urologist Professor Angel Garcia Fernandez discussed with Professor Peter Petros, who was the discoverer of the stress incontinence operation in which he had cured millions of women of incontinence.

The question to be answered was simple…*"Is there some way in which this discovery, of how the adult female pelvic floor works, can be applied to bed wetting children?"*

The answer is now in your hands, in this book, and is available to parents around the world, as well as doctors, specialists and others.

No more false, misleading information, or old wives tales. We now have scientific tests and results that can lead this health issue to the forefront, with real life changing statistics and results.

The answer to the questions these two international experts posed each other had to be non-surgical. Nobody wants a little boy or girl to undergo an operation.

Enter Dr. Patricia Skilling, a one-time colleague and collaborator of Professor Petros in his incontinence work with adult women. Dr. Skilling had devised a natural muscle pelvic floor exercise regime which had been effective in women suffering incontinence. Dr. Skilling's method of exercise was discussed by Professors Petros and Fernandez, but the problem was that, as published, it wasn't directly applicable to children.

So returning home, Professor Petros consulted with Dr. Skilling, and a simplified regime was instituted. This included ten full squats morning and evening, PLUS adopting a 'squatting culture' during the day. This consisted simply of asking the child never to bend down from the waist to pick something up, but instead to squat down, to pick up the toy or whatever, and then stand. Also, to have them try and do all their activities such as playing with toys in a squatting position, rather than a sitting position.

When Professor Fernandez undertook a research study with a large number of bed wetting children, it was anticipated that there would be a significant improvement in all pelvic floor symptoms. But the results of an 80% cure after four months of squats, in such a large group of youngsters, both boys and girls, was well beyond the expectations of the doctors. However, looked at in the context that these children were still in full-steam-ahead collagen creation mode to develop their bones, ligaments and tissues, all of which required collagen, the results are perfectly explainable. The doctors' delight, as well as the children's parents and the kids themselves, was overwhelming.

How Bedwetting Occurs

Now we need to go into a bit of anatomy. It will help explain why bed wetting occurs at night; and it's nothing to do with a full bladder or forgetfulness. It's all to do with geometry.

At night, the pelvic muscles referring to diagram 1.2 (large pink arrows) relax. As the patient sleeps, the bladder fills and expands downwards under the force of gravity 'G.' If the ligaments 'L' (purple lines) are weak, the base of the bladder with its nerve endings 'N' expands downwards. This stretching stimulates 'N' to send impulses 'O' (green) to the brain to activate the emptying reflex.

The brain sends down blocking impulses 'C' (red) to block the 'O' impulses.

A tug of war begins. When 'O' becomes more powerful, the emptying reflex is activated, and the child wets the bed.

What the exercises devised by Dr. Skilling do is to strengthen the 3 muscles (large pink arrows). These pull on the ligaments 'L' to strengthen them by the production of new collagen.

DIAGRAM 1.2

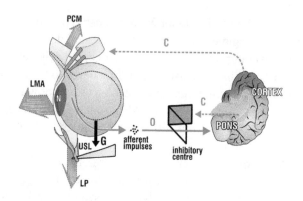

And the Ones Who Weren't Cured?

Let's look at the situation before these squatting exercises were discovered. The parents were told, and quite correctly so, that most children would be cured as they grew older and certainly, most would be cured once they had passed puberty. So any deficiencies from the squatting regime would necessarily fall into this category and it could be expected that most of the children who fail the squatting regime would improve or be cured by the time puberty passes.

At least as regards the female, once they had passed a certain age, help is at hand in the form of strengthening the weak ligaments by insertion of a tape in the exact position of the ligaments as in the 5,000,000 women who were cured of stress incontinence, either in the front or the back ligaments.

IMPORTANT

It is critical that these squatting exercises are performed twice daily without fail for a full 4 months. In order to ensure this happens it's advisable to keep a record on a calendar or diary. Please remember, it takes time for the exercises to induce the collagen to get into the ligament in order to strengthen it. Also, as collagen is replaced and replenished every 3 months, the exercises must become a daily routine, a habit to continue for many years.

What Exercises Can Your Child Do?

We cannot emphasize enough the importance of **ongoing** regular squats to strengthen the three automatic muscles, morning and night. Squatting twice daily is the most direct exercise to strengthen the pelvic floor and to create new collagen. It should become a daily habit.

Remember, from birth to their early 20's is the collagen-creation phase of their body, building up muscles, tissues, ligaments, bones. Those beyond middle-age are in the collagen-loss phase of their lives. They stoop, bend, even shrink in size.

The problem is people in Western societies have a no squatting culture. They bend from the waist when picking up objects. In contrast, children in Eastern and African cultures squat down to play as do adults when doing household tasks. We know from scientific studies that women from such cultures develop very strong pelvic ligaments and tissues.

Try and develop a squatting culture. At the very least, please remember, every time you need to pick something up, squat down to do it…don't bend!

How Can a Parent Convince a Child to Do These Vital Exercises Morning and Night, Sometimes for Years?

All kids like routine, but few like boring exercises. So why not turn the exercises into a game? **Each child will respond to a different game. The key principle is squatting, the more the better**. And you should vary them to retain your child's interest.

We have made a few suggestions below, such as when playing with their pet, they should squat, and not bend down, like this…

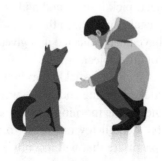

When watching tv or playing with toys, get them to squat and not sit. The more they squat, the more they're exercising the pelvic floor muscles which control their waste outlets. And the more efficient these muscles become, the sooner they'll stop involuntary peeing and pooping.

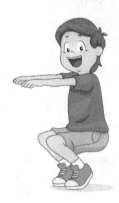

Game One – The Bunny (or Kangaroo) Hop

This is a fun game which any kid aged 2 or 3 upwards can play.
In your lounge room, or on the pathway of the house, lay down ten small objects in a long row. They could be buttons or coins, matchbox cars or something small.

Now start your daughter or son at the beginning of the row, facing towards the objects. Tell him or her to squat down, and hop (jump) to the first one. Pick it up and stand up to give it to mommy or daddy. Now squat down again and hop to the next object…just two or three hops. Grasp the next little object, pick it up, stand and give it to mommy or daddy. Now squat down again and hop to the next object…and on and on until all ten objects have been collected and given to a parent.

At the end of the row of little objects, when the 10th has been collected and given, then a reward such as a sticker can be presented for good work…collect, say, 14 stickers by the end of the week (meaning seven successful exercise regimes in the morning and seven in the afternoon) and the reward could be a small toy or a visit to a mall or park or something you deem appropriate that will incentivize your child.

Game Two – Pat-a-Cake

Remember the game Pat-a-Cake? That's where you face a friend, and clap hands; then hand slap the friend's opposite hand...your right against their left. Then back to clapping. It's from an ancient nursery rhyme...

"Pat-a-cake, pat-a-cake, baker's man.
Bake me a cake as fast as you can
Pat it, and prick it, and mark it with 'B'
And put it in the oven for Baby and me!"

You could play this with your son or daughter, while they're squatting.

Squat down (yes, you'll have to squat as well*) and play Pat-a-Cake. Then stand. Then squat and slap alternative hands. Then stand. Then squat again, and clap hands.

The child or you could make up variations. There could be a reward if the hand clapping or slapping is conducted successfully or perhaps playing with your child may be rewarding enough.

There's also a major reward for the mother who plays this game with her child. By squatting you are exercising the key muscles in your pelvis, you're strengthening them to help prevent the possibility of incontinence and leakage later on in their lives, more as they approach late middle age, and when women approach or pass menopause. So everybody benefits.

Game Three – Push The Ball

Place a ball on the ground. Get your child to squat down and have to push the ball from a squatting position across the room to a corner or across the backyard. Now they have to stand, walk to the ball and when they reach it, squat down again and push the ball to another point in the room or outside. Continue this ten times in the morning, and ten times at night, and that's what's required to stop his or her bedwetting.

But remember that you have to continue the exercises to maintain the strength of the muscles. And of course, you can vary it by encouraging your son or daughter to push their favorite wheeled toy.

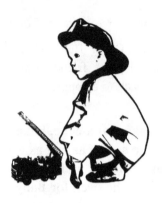

The Similarities Between Children and Adults

Some children find that they can't hold on sufficiently during the day to get to the toilet in time before they wet themselves. This condition is common in adults and is called urge incontinence. The cause is similar to bedwetting but slightly different in that the muscles can't stretch the organs sufficiently during the day to support the signaling mechanism to the brain for activation of emptying reflex.

Again, the treatment is the same...a minimum of ten squats in the morning and at night PLUS adopt a 'squatting culture.' Because the mechanisms for the bowel are very similar, if a child has problems containing the bowel, the same regime is suggested, a minimum of 10 squats morning and evening.

Some children have both bedwetting at night and incontinence during the day. Again, the treatment is the same.

Potential Psychological Damage to the Child

Often the parents will castigate the child who wets during the day because they are told by the well-meaning doctor they consult with, that it's the child's failing because he or she simply is too busy concentrating on other things and forgets to go to the toilet.

Of course, we have a very different point of view, which is that Nature has evolved a system that is perfect, that can contain large volumes of urine during the day as the bladder is remarkably accommodating to large volumes of urine – it simply expands like a balloon. So, the problem isn't in the bladder's volume, but in the inability of the muscles and ligaments to support and to close the emptying tube. Remember that during the day, most kids can hold on for hours without going to the toilet, until they realize, often suddenly, that they have to go. The same happens during the night. The bladder fills and expands, and in most cases, in the morning, allows the child to pass a large volume of urine. But in kids who wet their beds, or leak during the day, it is NOT forgetfulness, carelessness or inattention that causes them to have these mishaps, It's because their muscles are not strong enough to enable the ligaments to keep the opening of their waste tubes closed. Which is the focus of this book on how to strengthen the muscles and ligaments against which they pull.

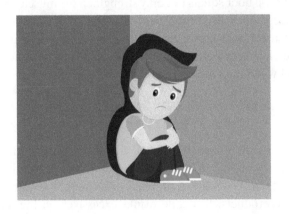

We have found that even the most rational of parents become frustrated and will blame the child for not paying attention during the day, or for not going to the toilet or drinking too much at night. This can unsettle a child's mental equilibrium. It's bad enough when the child is ridiculed at school by his or her classmates as a wee baby or poo baby. Children can be very cruel. There is a need for every child to be a comfortable, harmonious and compliant member of his or her peer group, a need which is essential for a child's well-being. Nobody wants to be an outlier and certainly not an exile from the group.

As we saw in the two diagrams earlier in this book, when, children are standing up, the organs in both boys and girls are basically supported by the muscles as well as the ligaments. However, when the child lies down to sleep, the muscles, instead of being horizontal, become vertical, and so the bladder has to rely on the ligaments to stop it distending downwards during sleep. In a normal patient, the ligaments support the bladder as it fills. If the ligaments are weak, they can't support the bladder as it distends downwards under the force of gravity. It is this stretching downwards which can activate the stretch receptors to give a signal to the brain to activate the emptying reflex, which is called the micturition reflex.

The first action of the micturition reflex is to relax the forward muscle, which is compressing the emptying tube, the urethra, from behind. When the bladder reaches a certain volume, this relaxation of the forward muscle allows the back muscles to open out the bladder neck. This further stimulates the emptying reflex, and the child wets the bed. The pelvic floor squats not only strengthen the muscles to keep the urethra closed, they also (importantly) strengthen the ligaments, so the muscles can contract more strongly to keep the urethral tube closed. A stronger ligament better supports the bladder when the patient is asleep and when the muscles are relaxed.

Does Limiting a Child's Fluid Intake Help Control His or Her Bedwetting?

The way the kidney words is that it filters the waste products from the body every minute of every hour whether the person is awake or asleep. So there is always a minimal urine output required to clear these waste products. If a child drinks excessively in the hours prior to sleeping, more urine will be produced than the minimum. However, only if a child is subjected to extreme deprivation of fluids would there be further decrease in urine output below the required normal, and probably not very much difference at that, as it would be extremely difficult for a very thirsty child to go to sleep.

What if a Child Has Difficulty in Evacuating the Bladder or the Bowel (Constipation)?

Another discovery of the Integral System by Professor Petros, dating from 1999 onwards, was that the mechanisms for opening the emptying tube of the bladder, the urethra, and the emptying tube of the bowel, the anus, were almost identical. The back muscles of the pelvis pulls down against the ligaments to open the back wall of the urethra and the anus. Think of it like water going through a garden hose. If the diameter of the hose is very narrow, there has to be a large amount of pressure to push the water through; whereas a large diameter hose allows the water to run through freely. In children and adults, the body makes it easier to empty the bladder and the bowel by pulling against the ligaments to open out the back wall of the tube to make it larger before evacuation starts.

If the ligaments are loose, then the muscles are too weak to open out the tube. The patient may have difficulty emptying the bladder in that it has a slow stream which stops and starts; or the patient can have difficulty in opening the bowel. This explains why in many constipated children, the feces may be small and narrow like rabbit stools. Again, if the patient is young, then the squatting exercises will not only strengthen the muscles which pull open the back wall of the emptying tubes, but it will strengthen the ligaments against which the muscles contract.

In short, the same pelvic exercises which work for the bladder and the bedwetting, should also improve the emptying of the bladder and the bowel.

CHRONIC PELVIC PAIN AFTER THE BEGINNING OF A YOUNG GIRL'S PERIODS

This sometimes happens in young girls. If it does, it is within a year or two after the establishment of her periods. Again, as part of Professor Petros' discovery of the Integral System, it was realized that there are special collections of nerves in the pelvis, which are supported by the back ligaments as they enter the uterus.

Think of it in terms of a bus station, where all the nerves of the pelvis (the buses) come into the station. These are nerves situated at the entrance to the vagina, near the anus, near the tailbone, the lower abdomen, next to the urethra and even the pelvic muscles. The 'bus station' is supported from below by the back ligaments. If the back ligaments are loose, the central complex of nerves (the bus station) remains unsupported and is dragged down by the force of gravity or the weight of the organs above it during the day. The pain is felt in all the areas where the 'buses' or nerves, come from, which have already been mentioned. This is called referred pain.

How Can This Be Proven?

Insert a large menstrual tampon to support the ligaments, and in at least half of the patients, there will be an improvement of their pain. This can also improve other symptoms dependent on these ligaments such as bladder emptying problems, urgency, and getting up at night… nocturia.

So How Do We Treat These Symptoms in Young Women?

Though only 14 or 15 years of age, they are still very much in collagen formation mode. Again, simple squatting is recommended, basic pelvic floor exercises are needed to strengthen the muscles and the ligaments. Or using a rubber Fit Ball instead of a chair is also a good technique as it strengthens the pelvic, abdominal and back muscles in a low-key way without the young woman realizing what's actually going on.

CASE HISTORIES

**Parents, and their children, find bed wetting somewhat
isolating. Unlike virtually every other disease or ailment in kids,
bed wetting is the one which is rarely talked about in public.**

Why? Because there's considerable embarrassment by adults and kids to admit that their child can't hold it in. It's as if the parent or child believes that it's their failing as people; because society, including almost every doctor and nurse, still thinks that the youngster has some agency and control over their involuntary wetting or pooing, as if they just need to control themselves – even when deeply asleep – in order to cure the ailment.

If there's ONE thing that this book has helped you understand, it's surely that bed wetting in kids is because of weak pelvic floor muscles. Not in all kids, but in a significant minority. Strengthen the muscles, and the problem should disappear.

In order to show you that you're not alone, here are some testimonials from parents who sought help for their own children.

They were written to Professor Angel Garcia Fernandez by South American parents of children who had been cured of bedwetting after four months of exercises.

Mr. and Mrs. Juarez

At the request of Dr. Garcia Fernandez, my wife and I wrote this little testimony about the improvement of our daughter Sofia who wet the bed almost every night. After the accomplishment of 4 months of simple exercises morning and night she improved. She can now go to sleep over with her friends. She is very happy.

Mrs. J. Arevalo

The whole family is very happy since our daughter did not wet the bed and improved her urgency to urinate and the losses she had during the day. Thanks to Doctor García Fernández and the man who proposed this treatment, Professor Peter Petros from Australia.

Mr. and Mrs. Andrade

Our son suffered for years from wetting the bed every night. It had great impact on his self-esteem and a lot of time and money was lost on psychologists and other specialists. Today he is a happy boy.

Thanks to those doctors, Professors Petros and Garcia Fernandez who did not rest in their efforts to devise new ways to cure our children.

Mr. and Mrs. White

It has been an awesome moment. A lot of time trying to correct urine losses and especially constipation in our 12 year old daughter. Four months of exercises made the problem disappear. Thanks so much to the doctors who made that possible.

Mr. and Mrs Canovas

We are Pilar's parents. Very happy with the treatment of enuresis of our son. It greatly improved his character and now he socializes with his friends. Thanks for so much Dr. Garcia Fernandez.

COMMENTS FROM A MEDICAL PRACTITIONER

As a clinical physician, I have treated many women who've suffered incontinence, more so in mothers and women approaching or post-menopausal. But many of the mothers undergoing pelvic floor exercises stated that they had had their bladder and bowel problems ever since they were children.

The fact that it had been a lifelong problem, and they had reported to have a 'weak' bladder since childhood was no impediment to improvement with the program. In most of them, their bladder had improved at puberty and they thought the problem was solved but were desperate when it returned after childbirth. And they slavishly followed the advice of physiotherapists and were religiously practicing the Kegel exercises, none of which solved their urgency, nocturia or pain problems.

So What Did That Tell Me About Incontinence... accidental, Untimely and Unwanted Wetting and Pooping...in Children?

That it's a devastating problem, and as you've read in this book by Professors Garcia Fernandez and Petros, children feel isolated and alone. In the worst cases, they are ostracized by their friends and this dramatically increases the dilemma, both for the parents and for the children themselves.

From a doctor's perspective, I found the stories about weak bladders in childhood quite fascinating. I've explored them thoroughly. The stories were, in fact, precisely the same as they were in adult patients. In the mild cases, they had an urge to go and empty their bladder. Sometimes as children they delayed and had to suddenly rush and often wet themselves before they arrived to the toilet. The more serious cases found that at a certain point, the urge came when they didn't have the time to go to the toilet and they wet their pants while they were standing there.

Another interesting fact was that sometimes, they may have had a brother or had known stories of an uncle or close relative who was like that as a child, which suggested to me that in some cases, these weak bladders may run in families.

Which brings me to myself and my family. My research and investigations over many years was brought home dramatically by my own family. First, my beautiful little grandson, aged six. His mother told me that her son, a little fellow with an amazing sense of humor, who laughed uproariously at school with his friends, but was sometimes wet and soiled himself to the point where his mum had to send him to school with a change of clothing. It was having an adverse psychological effect, with his friends calling him 'poo boy' and 'when are you going to get a nappy?' He began to become unusually morose and was easily embarrassed. These weren't normal emotions for this happy little boy.

The remarks of his classmates isolated and alienated him, and he slowly went from a truly well-adjusted little boy in the class to somebody who was constantly anxious, not only about laughing, but about everything, afraid to show his real personality in case he wet his pants.

His incontinence, both bladder and bowel, was sufficiently serious for my daughter to contact me. When I went to visit wanting to know more, I was horrified to see my daughter and her husband berated their son for 'not paying attention,' blaming him for wetting himself.

Now, both my daughter and her husband are superbly intelligent professional adults, yet they genuinely thought that my grandson had volition over wetting or soiling himself. I explained the mechanisms of the pelvic floor, that control of bladder and bowel was a reflex, meaning it was involuntary. Nobody, old or young had control over it. I told them about my patients, and how some of them had explained that 'weak' bladders ran in the family. She asked me why squatting would work on a youngster who played sports and was honed to muscular perfection. "What does squatting do, Mum?" she asked.

I told her that it wasn't just about strengthening the leg muscles. When somebody squats, the brain reflexly contracts the three pelvic floor muscles, which close the urethra and the anal canal. But the patient doesn't know that it's happening, unlike in the Kegel exercises, which are voluntary.

Then my daughter asked "How can I get a little boy to understand that he has to squat in order to help himself? You know kids...they'll do it for a day or two, and then forget about it."

I told her that I would explain to my grandson that as a cricket-mad fanatic, the exercises would make him into a top-class fielder and batsman. It would even improve his bowling. Not lies, exactly, but... well...you know...well-meaning fibs. I said that it should be reinforced by him doing the squatting exercises along with his little brother, as I believed that they were both destined to be brilliant cricketers, and these exercises would help them along their way.

I got him to practice squatting exercises which not only strengthened the muscles, but also the ligaments against which they contract. Then there was my little granddaughter from my husband's side of the family. Her problem was fairly mild by comparison, the sudden onset of urge from time to time to empty her bladder during the day. Her parents were told that the cause was intense concentration on her task at hand which made her forget to go to the toilet. Yet her sister, equally concentrated, had no such problem. Her older sister was well-organized, so they both began 10 squats every morning and night. The urge disappeared within a few weeks.

What about bed-wetting at night? We have had several surgical cures of women in their early twenties who had wet the bed at night as children and continued to do so as young adults. We repaired the front ligaments, exactly as we do for urinary stress incontinence, urine leakage on coughing. Squatting exercises had not helped these young women.

But will this work on every child? The best answer I can give to that is, irrespective of the age of the human being, the anatomy is the same.

So if every incontinent, bedwetting child does these squats, will this be an end to their problems? It's difficult to answer this question. Professors Garcia Fernandez and Petros have shown in a university trial that it works in 80% of cases. But clearly not all children will be improved; the best way to look at is that these squatting exercises strengthen the muscles which close the urethra and anus. Think of the pelvic floor as a series of muscles. Just as training an athlete will improve his or her ability to run or jump, so training the pelvic floor will improve the child's ability in the area of continence.

Unfortunately, simple as these methods appear to be, the drop-out rate of reasonably well-motivated adult women was 50%. I felt that asking my grandson to play with his toys in the squatting position rather than sitting down, at the age of six would have no chance of succeeding, if I hadn't told him it would improve his cricket and that by squatting, he could become a Grade 1 Cricketer. So, I enthused him with a daily routine morning and night of 10 squats each time.

And did it work? Oh yes! Within a week he was already better, and six weeks later...yes, just six weeks...he'd stopped all involuntary lapses. Whether he'll become an A-grade cricketer or not, I really don't know.

And there's another similar case which illustrates just how effective these exercises are. A very close friend who lives 100 miles north of me, phoned me one day for a chat; but I could tell from the stress in her voice that she was on the edge of tears. I asked her what was wrong, and she said that for the third time that week, she had to wash her four year old son's bed sheets because he'd soaked them during the night. And he'd soiled his pants with poop the previous day at kindergarten and had been shunned and teased by his young classmates. His teacher had been empathetic, given the child a pair of pants which the kindergarten kept on hand as spares for such emergencies, and wrapped up the offending pair in a plastic bag.

She'd been to her doctor who'd told her not to allow her son to drink anything after five in the evening, but it had made no difference. Now she was waiting for an appointment with a child psychologist.

While I had an appointment with Dr. Skilling about my own issue, I asked her about my friend's son. She suggested that the boy's mother should help him perform pelvic floor exercises. I phoned my friend and suggested that she do the exercises with her little boy while they watched cartoons on television in the afternoon. Every time a cartoon character jumped up into the air, or sat down, or bent over, her little boy watched carefully and used it as a moment for him to squat down, and then stand up.

He loved the game, which of course were exercises that would be good for strengthening the pelvic muscles.

After a week, the boy didn't lose control during the day, and after three weeks, his bed wetting had stopped at night.

It was amazing! And my friend immediately phoned up the child psychologist and cancelled the appointment. Then she phoned her doctor and told her about what she'd done and the miraculous effect it had had on her son. The doctor was surprised and happy to hear the news. He said that from now on, he'd tell his patients to do precisely what she'd done to help stop bed wetting.

AND A FINAL WORD FROM TWO PROFESSORS OF MEDICINE

We have been keen to stress a number of truly important points throughout this little book

Bed wetting doesn't affect a large percentage of older boys and girls, but for those it does affect, the consequences can cause a serious and life-impairing situation when it occurs. Because it's something kept secret from the outside world, the psychological damage to kids can be truly serious. It's NOT just a nuisance; it has to be dealt with.

Bed wetting is Nature telling the child to toughen up his or her pelvic muscles. It shouldn't be ignored or overlooked by a mother or father. The consternation it causes to kids can be truly devastating, especially in a boy's and girl's older years. It can ruin a social life, damage friendships and have long-term emotional consequences. This book gives YOU, the parent or grandparent, a way of dealing with it.

Bed wetting has nothing to do with the bladder, or a child's forgetfulness or lack of attention, or laziness, so punishment and threats are absolutely the wrong approach. Berating and threatening a child for wetting his bed is damaging to your relationship, and causing your child to feel guilt for something he or she can't help.

Bed wetting is caused by weak muscles and inadequate ligaments, both of which can be alleviated by the simple exercises we've shown you.

Regular exercises by squatting with your children will alleviate bed wetting in almost every case. And the wonderful thing about you, the mom or dad, doing the squatting exercises with the child, is that it may also help YOU in later life to avoid pelvic floor problems.

This self-help book has, hopefully, saved parents time and the expense of visits to doctors or specialists to cure a condition by simple, fun exercises.

But what if the exercises, done regularly and properly, don't work? Well, if after two or three months of twice daily squatting exercises monitored by you, and your son or daughter is still a regular bed wetter, then a visit to a pediatrician or pediatric urologist is probably advisable, just to check that everything is in proper working order. And one more thing. If you do go to a doctor, please remember to take this book with you.

We wish you good and continued health
for you and your family

Dr. Angel Garcia Fernandez
Dr. Peter Petros

STOP PRESS

At a meeting held recently in Gdansk, Poland for some 180 pediatricians, pediatric urologists and other doctors specializing in childhood incontinence, the latest 'research' into the field was presented. They were told that nocturnal enuresis – bed wetting – does not seem to be affected by drugs such as those used to reduce thirst. They also discussed research showing that children who wet their beds at night may have a somewhat impaired sense of smell.

According to the two authors of this book, this research is nonsensical and distracting. Professor Fernandez writes of a very recent case he has cured of a boy, aged six, who was a chronic retentive and whose incontinence presented as effort to go to the toilet and urgency. The poor child urinated irregularly and in pain. He was very constipated. Professor Fernandez urged the boy do to squatting exercises, and after only one week, the problem disappeared. He is now on a maintenance level of exercise. Dr. Fernandez said, "I have been seeing these patients for many years, and the exercises are an incredible advance in the application of the Integral Theory to bedwetting. They really truly are a miracle breakthrough."

The major treatment breakthroughs in this book may appear simple, but are based on a researched and thorough scientific program. We are reprinting the academic paper which first introduced this breakthrough in treatment to the world's pediatricians and general practitioners.

It is meant for doctors to read and understand, so please feel free to give this book to your treating physician so that he or she can read the paper we published in the Central European Journal of Urology, and gain a greater understanding of why this treatment is so effective.

CENTRAL EUROPEAN JOURNAL OF UROLOGY

A four month squatting-based pelvic exercise regime cures day/night enuresis and bowel dysfunction in children 7–11 years

Angel Garcia-Fernandez[1], Peter Emanuel Petros[2,3]

[1]Universidad Nacional de Córdoba, Department of Pediatric Surgery, Córdoba, Argentina,
[2]University of NSW Professorial, Department of Surgery, St Vincent's Hospital, Sydney, Australia
[3]School of Mechanical and Chemical Engineering, University of Western Australia, Perth, Australia

Citation: Garcia-Fernandez A, Petros PE. A four month squatting-based pelvic exercise regime cures day/night enuresis and bowel dysfunction in children 7–11 years. Cent European J Urol. 2018; doi: 10.5173/ceju.2020.0044 [Epub ahead of print]

Article history
Submitted: March 5, 2020
Accepted: June 28, 2020
Published online: July 20, 2020

Corresponding author
Peter Petros
31/29 Elizabeth Bay Rd.
NSW 2011 Elizabeth Bay
Australia
phone: +61 411 181 731
pp@ kvinno.com

Introduction In 2004 Patricia Skilling developed a new squatting-based pelvic floor rehabilitation method based on strengthening the three reflex pelvic muscles and ligaments hypothesized to control the closure and micturition reflexes. We adapted these methods to test our hypothesis that day/night enuresis was due to the inability of these muscles/ligaments to control an inappropriately activated micturition reflex.
Material and methods The trial commenced as a randomized control trial to be conducted over 4 months, but was converted to a prospective trial at 4 weeks by order of the Ethics Committee. A total of 48 children, 7.6 ±2.5 years, 34 females, 14 males, had strictly supervised exercises twice daily, 10 squats, 10 bridge, fitball exercises involving proprioception exercises with surface perineal electromyogram (EMG) once a week.
Eligibility criteria was daytime urine leakage plus night-time bedwetting. Exclusion criteria was refusal to sign consent forms. Assessment was done by intention to treat. The criterion for cure was complete dryness.
Results At 1st review (4 weeks) 12/24 in the treatment group reported total cure of wetting; 41/48 children (86%) were cured of both daytime/nighttime enuresis (p <0.001) at 4 months. There were no adverse events. Secondary outcomes were concomitant cure of constipation, fecal incontinence, urinary retention as predicted by the underlying integral theory of incontinence.
Conclusions We believe our methods accelerated normal childhood strengthening of muscles/ligaments which control inappropriate activation of the micturition reflex which we hypothesize is the basis for daytime/nighttime enuresis. This is a simple treatment, but it needs validation by others.

Key Words: feasibility ◊ general anesthesia ◊ proximal ureter stone ◊ spinal anesthesia ◊ reterorenoscopy

INTRODUCTION

Nocturnal enuresis or 'bedwetting' syndrome represents an important percentage of the daily consultation of the pediatrician/pediatric urologist. An estimated 15–20% of children at 5 years of age wet the bed [1]. Little is known about the pathophysiology or how to treat it [1], other than it may be a genetic and heterogeneous disorder [2, 3, 4]. Different specialties consider the topic from their own viewpoint, particularly psychologists and psychiatrists who see the problem as a behaviour disorder.

The Standardization Committee of the International Society for Pediatric Continence [5] specifically avoided pathogenesis and treatment in its 2016 publication. The committee separated day and night incontinence thus: "Intermittent incontinence that occurs while awake is termed daytime incontinence. When intermittent incontinence occurs exclusively during sleeping periods, it is termed enuresis"; and

"Symptoms are classified according to their relation to the storage and/or voiding phase of bladder function, but terminology used for lower urinary tract (LUT) symptoms will focus on descriptive rather than quantitative language."

Another vision and the basis of this paper, is the 1990 Integral Theory of Female Urinary Incontinence which states that bladder incontinence is a consequence of lax suspensory ligaments due to collagen changes therein [6]; symptom control is by three involuntary directional muscle forces which act against pubourethral and uterosacral/cardinal ligaments (CL/USL) to close urethral and anal tubes, Figure 1, Video 1; to open them for micturition by selective relaxation of a forward muscle, (arrow, Figure 2), and control of the micturition reflex by a central and peripheral neurological feedback system [7], Figure 2. In this context, 'overactive bladder' (OAB) is mainly an uncontrolled activation of the micturition reflex [8] expressed as urge incontinence during the day and nocturia at night. If ligaments are loose, the directional muscles which contract against them weaken; the muscles can no longer stretch the organs sufficiently to support the hydrostatic pressure of the urine (and feces) acting on the stretch receptors 'N', Figure 2; 'N' fire off afferents to the cortex at a lower bladder volume; if central control of the afferents (white arrow, fig 2) cannot stem the afferent flow, the micturition or defecation reflexes are activated and the adult (and child) perceives this as an urge to empty the bladder (or bowel) during the day; at night, nocturia. A fundamental aspect of pelvic symptoms is the 'iceberg phenomenon' [9] where there is one main presenting symptom, in this work, nocturnal enuresis; the other symptoms such as daytime wetting, constipation, bladder emptying problems are 'below the surface' and have to be specifically sought out by direct questioning.

Proofs of the theory to date have been largely surgical: observation of symptom fate following ligament repair. Examples: cure of stress urinary incontinence (SUI), by the midurethral sling [10] with a tape placed in the position of the pubourethral ligament (estimated 10,000,000 operations to date). Not so well known is cure of organ prolapse and pelvic symptoms by tapes placed in the cardinal and uterosacral ligaments [11–16]. Even less well known are Patricia Skilling's squatting-based pelvic floor exercises (PFE) in a premenopausal adult population [17, 18]. These work by strengthening the 3 involuntary pelvic muscles and the ligaments they contract against; the PFEs achieved a greater than 50% improvement in urge, nocturia, stress urinary incontinence and bowel symptoms in 70–90% of premenopausal women [17, 18]. Some women were nulliparous and had

nocturnal enuresis as children, suggesting, perhaps, a congenital etiology. It was this part of her results which inspired this study.

We hypothesized

1. Nocturnal enuresis and daytime incontinence in children may be caused by congenital muscle/ligament weakness destabilizing control of the micturition reflex.

2. Nocturnal enuresis is the adult equivalent of nocturia, except that the children do not wake.

3. As children are in a collagen creation phase for their tissues, ligaments and bones, the squatting-based exercises would strengthen the 3 directional forces which open and close bladder and bowel, Figures 1&2, and create new collagen to reinforce pubourethral and cardinal/uterosacral ligaments to reverse the urinary and fecal dysfunctions as per the pelvic floor exercise studies [17, 18].

The primary aim was to test these hypotheses with an randomized control trial (RCT) with squatting-based exercises against placebo. The secondary aim was to test the 'iceberg' concept of co-occurrence of other bladder and bowel symptoms such as constipation, fecal incontinence, emptying symptoms by monitoring their fate.

MATERIAL AND METHODS

The study was carried out at the Integral Institute of Pelvic Floor in the city of Córdoba – Argentina, after approval of the work plan by the Ethics Committee of CEIS Oulton, Instituto Oulton, affiliation, Faculty of Medical Sciences of the UNC under the supervision of the first author AFG. IRB approval by the ACTA B-345 Registro Provincial De Investigacion En Salud. **Initial study design.** A randomized control study with two arms, squatting-based pelvic floor exercises and a placebo arm. The study was performed at the Instituto Integral de Piso Pélvico Cordoba Argentina. Declaration of Helsinki and CONSORT guidelines were followed. Recruitment period: 26.8.2019 to 26.12.2019.

Participants. Forty-eight children were entered into the study by their parents.

Inclusion criteria were male and female patients from 6 to 10 years of age with night-time enuresis (bedwetting) plus daytime wetting. Written informed consent from parents for the patients included in the study including permission to publish the results.

Exclusion criteria were patients whose parents did not accept informed consent.

The presenting symptom in all 48 children was nocturnal enuresis. Other symptoms recorded were

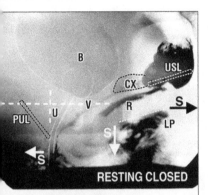

RESTING CLOSED

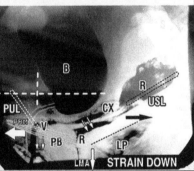

STRAIN DOWN

Figure 1. *Three directional muscle actions* pull against pubo-urethral (PUL) and uterosacral (USL) suspensory ligaments Broken lines represent bony vertical and horizontal co-ordinates . Radioactive dye has been inserted into the bladder 'B', vagina 'V', rectum 'R' and levator plate 'LP'
Upper xray image Three slow twitch muscle forces 'S' maintain continence.
Lower xray image Urethral closure On straining, three fast twitch muscles pull forwards and backwards against the pubo-rethral ligaments 'PUL' (arrows) and downwards against the uterosacral ligaments 'USL' (downward arrow). The downward vector 'LMA' pulls down the anterior border of LP to 'kink' the urethra at bladder neck.
Anorectal closure PRM contracts forwards. The backward vector LP stretches the rectum 'R' back to tension it; the downward vector 'LMA'rotates 'R' to close the anorectal angle. Forward vector = m.pubococcygeus; backward vector = m.levator plate 'LP'; downward vector = m. conjoint longitudinal muscle of the anus 'LMA'.

daytime wetness, constipation, consistency and frequency of stools (Bristol classification), urinary tract infection, urge symptoms during the day, bladder emptying problems. Also recorded were age; residence (urban/rural); family situation: couples with stable union or unstable unions; change of residency in the previous 6 months; socio-economic level: low, medium, high; retention and urgency: whether the child was undergoing perineal maneuvers to retain urine and if urine was urgent to urinate; medication: none, past treatment with desmopressin and / or imipramine. No medication was administered during the study, except antibiotics if urinary infection was detected.
Urinary infection was diagnosed with positive urine culture to determine causal germ and treatment.

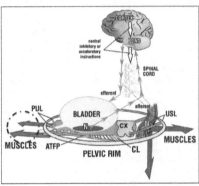

Figure 2. *Binary control of bladder & bowel . Schematic 3D sagittal view.* System in normal closed mode. Like a trampoline, the organs are stretched and balanced by 3 opposite muscle forces (red arrows), contracting against PUL (pubourethral ligaments) and USL (uterosacral ligaments). Afferent impulses (small green arrows) originating from stretch receptors 'N' travel to the cortex. They are routinely reflexly suppressed cortically (white arrows). When required, the cortex activates the defecation and micturition reflexes for evacuation: the forward muscles relax, pubococcygeus for urethra (broken circle), puborectalis for anus (not shown); this allows the posterior muscles (arrows) to unrestrictedly open out the posterior wall of anus and urethra (broken white lines) just prior to bladder/ rectal evacuation by smooth muscles contraction (spasm). If PUL or USL are loose, the muscles contracting against them (red arrows) weaken. Urethra/anus cannot be closed (incontinence), opened (emptying problems) or organs stretched to support 'N', ('urge incontinence).

CX = cervix; CL = cardinal ligament; ATFP = arcus tendineus fascia pelvis.

Constipation was defined as periods of 2 or more days without evacuation, as well as quality of the stools on the (hard or soft) Bristol scale.

Bladder emptying symptoms were confirmed by urine flowmetry and simultaneous computerized urine volume per second, duration of urination and activity of perineal floor with EMG perineal contact electrodes connected to an electromyograph (Medware®) brand with Ecud XP 5.0® and Ace XP 5.0® software.

The 3rd exercise, kinesiotherapy was carried out in the laboratory, the objective being for the child to identify the muscles that contract during exercises.

Psychological evaluation was performed if considered relevant. It provided information about the different profiles of children and their families to achieve a better approach to each patient. The nutritionist's analysis delved into the hygienic-dietary aspects necessary to contribute to the improvement of constipation.

Randomization and masking. All 48 children in the study had daytime and nightly bedwetting, Table 1. Details were taken by a nurse who explained there was a new treatment and asked if they would participate in a trial which was explained. On agreement a consent form was signed. Meanwhile, 24 printed copies of each treatment were randomly placed into sealed opaque envelopes gathered into a box and shuffled thoroughly by a 2nd (blinded) person. The box was taken to the outpatient clinic. As each child entered the trial, two envelopes were taken from the box and placed on the desk. One envelope was chosen by the parent and the child was assigned to the trial arm indicated in the envelope. The next child was assigned according to the remaining envelope and so on. Care was taken so every step of the trial, randomization, intervention and assessment, was carried out by a different person, each person blinded from the other.

Treatment arm protocol: involved 3 types of exercises. The parents were directly instructed how to do the exercises at the clinic and were also given explanatory videos.
1. Ten squats morning and evening at home.
2. Ten bridge exercises morning and evening at home.
3. Fitball exercises involving pelvic anteversion and retroversion once a week in the clinic laboratory which involved proprioception exercises with surface perineal EMG. The rationale for this was that surface EMG helped compliance of the children to the exercises. It improved the proprioception and they assumed it as something playful.

The placebo arm protocol: the children ran 50 meters in the morning and also at night.
Monitoring was with diaries.

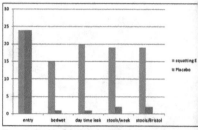

Figure 3. *Graphic of the first part of the trial. Symptom improvement at one month*

Outcomes, Table 1

Forty-eight children were studied; 96% carried out 4 months of exercises and completed the follow-up. Two were lost to the study. There were no adverse events.

Primary outcomes (intention to treat)

41/48 children were cured of both daytime/nighttime enuresis (p <0.001).
Criterion for cure was complete dryness at 4 months review.

Secondary outcomes

32 (68%) had constipation with 92% cured (P<0.001); 9 (19%) soiling (all cured), 6 females (12%) a history of urinary tract infection, 15 (31%) had bladder emptying difficulties confirmed by 'staccato wave' on fluometry and post-void residual urine (PVR). Cure was confirmed in all 15 by ultrasound post-void residual (PVR).

Mean age was 7.6 ±2.5 years, 34 females and 14 males. The vast majority of these children were from urban areas (78%) and the family situation was stable in 96% of the children. These children, mostly, had a medium socio-economic level (64%), an 18% lower class and 18% upper class. Demographics had no influence on outcomes.

The presenting symptom in every case was bedwetting. All other symptoms were obtained by specific interrogation. The main symptomatic results are detailed in Table 1.

Both arms of the RCT results were assessed at 4 weeks, Figure 3, by an external assessor whose opinion was validated by the parent of the child and entered into the clinical notes, stamped and dated.

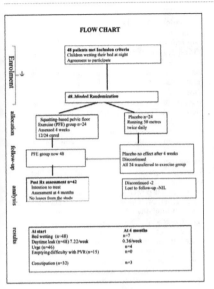

FLOW CHART

Enrolment

48 patients met inclusion criteria
Children wetting their bed at night
Agreement to participate

allocation

48 blinded Randomization

Squatting-based pelvic floor
Exercise (PFE) group n=24
Assessed 4 weeks
12/24 cured

Placebo n=24
Running 50 metres
twice daily

follow-up

PFE group now 48

Placebo no effect after 4 weeks
Discontinued
All 24 transferred to exercise group

analysis

Post Rx assessment n=42
Intention to treat
Assessment at 4 months
No losses from the study

Discontinued -2
Lost to follow-up -NIL

results

At start	At 4 months
Bed wetting (n=48)	n=7
Daytime leak (n=48) 7.22/week	0.36/week
Urge (n=46)	n=4
Emptying difficulty with PVR (n=15)	n=0
Constipation (n=32)	n=3

In the exercise group, 12/24 were entirely dry. In the control arm, there was no change. All children remained wet. At this point, the IRB committee ordered that the RCT be stopped, the placebo arm transferred to the exercise arm and the trial continued as a prospective trial. No child complained of pelvic pain and there was no stress urinary incontinence. Transperineal ultrasound did not show any abnormal perineal descent or any bladder neck funnelling.

Treatment prior to the trial 14 patients had some medication (Desmopressin10, Imipramine 3. oxybutynin 1), with no significant effect. 19 consulted with psychologists. Only some found some degree of impact on their self-esteem. There was no depression. There was no medication given.

10% of patients had urinary infections and 68% were considered constipated.

Gathering and assessment of the results

Each of the variables obtained upon admission (Table 1) were followed for a period of 4 months: at 2 weeks, 4 weeks and 4 months, each stage by a separate blinded assessor. At 4 months, the results were assessed again by a separate blinded assessor and validated in writing on the clinical notes by the parent with a signed signature and a dated hospital stamp. Analysis was separately carried out. We found

a statistically significant difference (p <0.001), when comparing the number of urine samples per day at the beginning of the study, with those observed at 4 months of follow-up. The difference between study entry and after 2 weeks of treatment was also significant (p <0.001).

Wetting during the day was another variable studied. We found differences between the beginning of the study (p <0.001) and at two weeks; differences between the 2 weeks of the study and one month (p <0.001). There were no differences between the month of the study and the end (0.99).

Bedwetting at night: difference was significant with respect to the start parameters and the subsequent observations (p <0.001). Differences were found between the data obtained after 2 weeks of treatment and the month of treatment (p = 0.022) and between the month of treatment and follow-up after 4 months (0.003).

Evacuation habit: we observed that the number of depositions per week was increasing according to the progress of the treatment, there being significant differences between the beginning of the study and the first 2 weeks of the same (p <0.001), between the 2 weeks of the study and the month of the same (p <0.001) with no differences between the 1 and 4 months of follow-up (p = 0.19).

Consistency of the stool: we found that significantly (p <0.001), the feces became softer between the beginning and the 2 weeks of treatment and this stool softening continued during the study, observing differences between the 2 weeks of treatment and the month of treatment (p = 0.006) and between the month of treatment and 4 months of follow-up (p <0.001).

Statistics

The statistical analysis for the evaluation of patients with enuresis and its treatment was carried out with SAS software (SAS Institute, Inc., Cary, NC). The numerical variables were presented as means ± standard deviation and the continuous ones as percentages, the comparisons of the numerical variables were made with the student or Wilcoxon test, as appropriate and the nominal variables with chi-square or exact test of Fisher according to the characteristics of the population. The analysis of all the variables was done individually with simple and logistic regressions and jointly by means of multiple and logistic regressions. When the comparison was made in more than two groups, the analysis of variance (ANOVA) was used. Participants were included in primary analyses by intention to treat (n = 48).

Determination of the sample

It was obtained with an alpha of 0.05 and a beta of 0.30. The delta observed in previous studies was quite broad, which allowed us to obtain a power or power of 90% with the study of 48 patients.

DISCUSSION

Though started as an RCT, the transfer of the placebo arm to the experimental arm effectively altered this work to a one arm prospective trial. The muscle/ligament concepts driving this study are well outside the normal conceptual thinking and treatments of learned societies in the pediatric field [5]. The results were well beyond our expectations: 86% cure of nocturnal enuresis and daytime incontinence. We expected results similar to Patricia Skilling's reports in adults, 50% improvement in 60–70% of children at most. The secondary outcomes, Table 1, demonstrated the importance of understanding that pelvic symptoms in the child occur in predictable groupings, and like the 'iceberg' concept [9], one symptom is pre-eminent. Other symptoms are 'under the surface' and need to be exposed by specific interrogation, as they were in our study protocol.

Analysis of hypothesis validity

Hypothesis 1 "Nocturnal enuresis and daytime incontinence in children may be caused by congenital ligament weakness destabilizing control of the micturition reflex." It is clear from Figure 1 and Video 1 https://www.youtube.com/watch?v=3vJx2OvUYe0, that squatting -based exercises will strengthen the three directional muscle forces and the ligaments they contract against, pubourethral 'PUL' and uterosacral 'USL' ligaments. During micturition and defecation, the backward/downward posterior muscle forces (large arrows), Figure 2, contract against USL to pull open out the posterior wall of urethra and anorectum, broken lines. Opening the urethra Video 2 https://www.youtube.com/watch?v=eiF4G1mk6EA&feature=youtu.be or rectum Video 3 https://youtu.be/MS82AZoWn7U exponentially decreases the resistance to flow of urine and feces inversely by the 4th power of the tube radius (Poiseuille's Law) [19–22]. This law is essential to understanding why children cannot close their emptying tubes (incontinence) or open them (constipation, bladder emptying difficulties): even a minor degree of muscle/ligament weakness is sufficient to cause bladder and bowel symptoms. Conversely, even a minor degree of strengthening will have an exponentially positive effect on the symptoms, as noted in our study.

The videos show the directional muscle movements of the muscles activated by the closure and evacuation reflexes.
Video 1. (Adult) 2D transperineal ultrasound showing the 3 directional movements activated by straining down. What to look for: involuntary forward movement acting against PUL position at midurethra; backward movement acting against PUL; downward angulation of the anterior border of the levator plate (white) against position of USL.
Video 2. Micturition (Adult) What to look for: involuntary backward movement acting against PUL; downward angulation of the anterior border of the levator plate against position of USL. 'Spasm' of detrusor throughout the emptying.
Video 3. Defecation (Adult) What to look for: downward angulation of the anterior border of the levator plate against position of USL exactly as occurs during micturition. Opening out of the anorectal angle; feces 'sliding' down the posterior rectal wall.
Hypothesis 2 "Nocturnal enuresis is the adult equivalent of nocturia, except that the children do not wake". It was not possible to objectively test an activated micturition reflex in children while they were asleep. However, on the basis that an 86% cure of nocturnal enuresis by muscle/ligament strengthening gives a similar result to nocturia, cure rates achieved in adults by surgical and non-surgical ligament strengthening [17, 18], we felt the hypothesis was validated: strengthening the peripheral stretch receptors 'N', Figure 2. restores normality to the feedback control system to prevent inappropriate activation of the micturition reflex, expressed as daytime urge, nocturia, bedwetting.
Hypothesis 3 "Children are in a collagen creation phase for their tissues, ligaments and bones, the squatting-based exercises would strengthen the 3 directional forces which open and close bladder and bowel, Figures 1 and 2, and create new collagen to reinforce PUL and CL/USL ligaments to reverse the urinary and fecal dysfunction." There is ample evidence in the literature of collagenotrophic activity during exercise for both muscles and connective tissue [23, 24]. Type I collagen is known to adapt to physical activity, and biomarkers of collagen turnover indicate that synthesis can be influenced by a single intense exercise bout [25]. Our findings were consistent with such evidence, but they did not prove hypothesis.
Strengths of the study Its simplicity and virtually zero cost. If validated by others, it will change the management of nocturnal enuresis and other symptoms in children forever. It will also change the science away from the organ itself, to the muscles and ligaments which act coordinately to open and close the outlet tubes.

Weakness of the study Data from a single study location. Stopping of the RCT after one month.

Limitations If, as seems likely, the pathway to cure is collagenopoiesis, it follows that exercises must be diligently performed, preferably for life.

CONCLUSIONS

We believe our methods accelerated normal childhood strengthening of muscles/ligaments which control premature activation of the micturition reflex which we hypothesize is the basis for daytime/night-time enuresis. This is a simple treatment, but it needs validation by others.

ACKNOWLEDGMENTS
To Dr Patricia Skilling for her assistance in adapting her adult Pelvic Floor protocols to the needs of the children.

CONFLICTS OF INTEREST
The authors declare no conflicts of interest.

References

1. Moffat M. Nocturnal enuresis. Is there a rationale for treatment? Scan J Urol Nephol Suppl. 1994; 163: 55-67.

2. Hublin C, Kaprio J, Partinen M, Koskenvuo M. Sleep. Nocturnal enuresis cohort. 1998; 21: 579.

3. Bakwin H. The genetics of enuresis, In: I. Kolvin, R.C. Mac Keith & S.R. Meadow (eds). Bladder Control and Enuresis. Rutter M, Yule W & Graham P; 1973, pp. 73-77.

4. Hjalmas K, Arnold T, Bower W, et al. Nocturnal enuresis: an international evidence-based management strategy. J Urol. 2004; 171: 2545-2561.

5. Austin PF, Bauer SB, Bower W, et al. The standardization of terminology of lower urinary tract function in children and adolescents: Update report from the standardization committee of the International Children's Continence Society. Neurourol Urodyn. 2016; 35: 471-448.

6. Petros PE & Ulmsten U. An Integral Theory of female urinary incontinence. Acta Obst Gynecolo Scand. 1990; 69 (Suppl 153): 1-79.

7. Petros PE. Detrusor instability and low compliance may represent different levels of disturbance in peripheral feedback control of the micturition reflex. Neurourol Urodyn. 1999; 18: 81-91.

8. Petros PE & Ulmsten U. Bladder instability in women: A premature activation of the micturition reflex. Neurourol Urodyn. 1993; 12: 235-239.

9. Goeschen K. Role of uterosacral ligaments in the causation and cure of chronic pelvic pain syndrome. Pelviperineology. 2015; 34: 2-20.

10. Ulmsten U, Petros P, Intravaginal slingplasty (IVS): an ambulatory surgical procedure for treatment of female urinary incontinence. Scand J Urol Nephrol. 1995; 29: 75-82.

11. Petros PE, Swash M. The Musculoelastic Theory of anorectal function and dysfunction. J Pelviperineology. 2008; 27: 89-121.

12. Liedl B, Inoue H, Sekiguchi Y, et al. Update of the Integral Theory and System for Management of Pelvic Floor Dysfunction in Females European J of Urology EURSUP-738. Eur Urol Suppl. 2018; 17: 100-108.

13. Wagenlehner F, Muller-Funogea I, Perletti G, et al. Vaginal apical prolapse repair using two different sling techniques improves chronic pelvic pain, urgency and nocturia - a multicentre study of 1420 patients. Pelviperineology. 2016; 35: 99-104.

14. Petros P, Lynch W, Bush M. Surgical repair of uterosacral/cardinal ligaments in the older female using the tissue Fixation system improves symptoms of obstructed micturition and residual urine. Pelviperineology. 2015; 34: 112-116

15. Inoue, H Kohata Y, Sekiguchi Y, Kusaka T, Fukuda T, Monnma M. The TFS minisling restores major pelvic organ prolapse and symptoms in aged Japanese women by repairing damaged suspensory ligaments- 12-48 month data. Pelviperineology. 2015; 34: 79-83.

16. Liedl B, Goeschen K, Yassouridis A, et al. Cure of Underactive and Overactive Bladder Symptoms in Women by 1,671 Apical Sling Operations Gives Fresh Insights into Pathogenesis and Need for Definition Change. Urol Int. 2019; 103: 228-234.

17. Petros PE, Skilling PM. Pelvic floor rehabilitation according to the Integral Theory of Female Urinary Incontinence. First report. Eur J Obstet Gynecol Reprod Biol. 2001; 94: 264-269.

18. Skilling PM, Petros PE. Synergistic non-surgical management of pelvic floor dysfunction: second report. Int J Urogyne. 2004; 15: 106-110.

19. Bush MB, Petros PEP, Barrett-Lennard BR. On the flow through the human urethra. Biomechanics. 1997; 30: 9,967-969.

20. Petros PE, Swash. M Directional muscle forces activate anorectal continence and defecation in the female. J Pelviperineology. 2008; 27: 94-97.

21. Bush M, Petros P, Swash M, Fernandez M, Gunnemann. Defecation 2: Internal anorectal resistance is a critical factor in defecatory disorders. Tech Coloproctol. 2012; 16: 445-450.

22. Petros PEP, Bush M. A Feedback Control System Explains Clinical and Urodynamic Bladder Instability in The Female. Pelviperineology. 2016; 35: 90-93.

23. Miller BF, Hansen M, Olesen JL, et al. Tendon collagen synthesis at rest and after exercise in women. J Appl Physiol. 2007; 102: 541-546.

24. Miller BF, Olesen JL, Hansen M, et al. Coordinated collagen and muscle protein synthesis in human patella tendon and quadriceps muscle after Exercise. J Physiol. 2005; 567: 1021-1033.

25. Langberg H, Skovgaard D, Asp S, et al. Time pattern of exercise-induced changes in type i collagen turnover after prolonged endurance exercise in humans Calcif Tissue Int. 2000; 67: 41-44. ▪

CPSIA information can be obtained
at www.ICGtesting.com
Printed in the USA
LVHW080033040920
665076LV00006B/364